Also by Dr. Stenbeck

Available from the usual on-line source

Books
Healing Yourself -- The Holistic Approach
  [An introduction to Holistic Self-healing.]

Heal Yourself Right Now!
  [The Seven Priority Organ Levels for
  effective Nutritional/Holistic Treatment of
  all organs.]

The 22 Unique Body Types
  (for Health and Weight Loss)

Q & A to Identify Your Body Type (Booklet)
  [Individual Type booklets are also available

Booklets
(Step-by-step instructions on healing yourself)

  #1 Start Healing with Positive Thinking
  #2 Mastering Positive Feelings for Health!
  #3 Spiritual Balance and Your Healing

The Lipopheric Body Type

Representing one of the 22 Body Types first described by Victor Rocine around 1900

The Senator Chris Christie, Rosie O'Donnell Celebrity Body Type

For Kaye,
there at the beginning with Doc Severn,
and for Liberty,
continuing the holistic healing journey...

About the Author

Educated in New Zealand and in the U.S.A., Dr. Stenbeck attained B.Sc. (NZ), M.S., and D.C. degrees. His holistic healing methods have been profiled in magazines (Esquire, McLean's, Playgirl, the Atlanta Constitution), and on TV in the USA and in Canada. He was the main contributor to the Warner Book, _The Eye/Body Connection_ by Jessica Maxwell that focused on the holistic healing relationships between the iris structure and organ genetics.

In the 1970-80's he was elected Fellow, Royal Society of Health, London; Fellow, American Association of Chemists; Member, American Association of Clinical Chemists; and Affiliate, Royal Society of Medicine, London. He studied naturopathy and Body Types with Dr. Bernard Jensen and Dr. Clifford Severn, and has practiced in medical partnerships where patients received the joint benefits of medical and holistic healing.

He is a member of Self-Realization Fellowship. To receive advice on any health issue from a holistic viewpoint, or to receive help with your body type, see his web site: *DrStenbeck.net*

———

Contents

* * *

The Lipopheric Body Type and Food Guide   1

The 22 Body Types: Celebrity Examples

This Booklet contains the Lipopheric type. See <u>The 22 Unique Body Types</u> for all type descript-ions.]

Thin Types

Atrophic	*Woody Allen / Audrey Hepburn* *Stan Laurel / Calista Flockheart*
Exesthesic	*Cher / Sarah Jessica Parker* *(Female type only)*
Marasmic	*President Obama / Princess Diana* *James Stewart / Kate Blanchard*
Neurogenic	*J.K. Simmons / Joan Rivers* *Jon Cryer / Marin Hinle*
Pathoferic	*(No celebrity males)* *Blythe Danner / Gwyneth Paltrow*
Sillevitic	*David Bowie / Shirley MacLaine* *Rod Stewart / Carol Channing*

Muscle Types

Calciferic	*Michael Jordan / Angelica Huston* *Abraham Lincoln / Grace Jones*
Carbogenic	*George Clooney / Lady Gaga* *Pres. G. Bush, Jr. / Meg Ryan*
Desmogenic	*Marlon Brando / Loni Anderson* *Daniel Craig / Tina Turner*
Eldic	*Ross Perot / Hillary Clinton* *Peter Falk / Sigourney Weaver*
Medeic	*Gary Oldman / Madonna* *John Hurt / Marlene Deitrich*
Myogenic	*Pres. Bill Clinton / Sharon Stone* *Pres. John Kennedy / Julia Roberts*
Nervimotive	*Frank Sinatra / Elizabeth Taylor* *Mark Wahlberg / Natalie Wood*
Nitropheric	*Ben Affleck / Ava Gardner* *Kirk Douglas / Kate Winslet*
Pallinomic	*Pres. Donald Trump /* *Attorney General Janet Reno* *Bill O'Reilly (Fox) / Jane Russell*

Fat Types

Barotic	*Robin Williams / 'Mrs.Doubtfire' Elton John / William Conrad*
Carboferic	*Bill Murray / Roseanne Billy Gardell / Melissa McCarthy*
Hydripheric	*John Goodman / Shelly Winters Wayne Knight / Jennifer Holliday*
Isogenic	*Einstein / Oprah Winfrey Phillip S .Hoffman / Queen Victoria*
Lipopheric	*Rush Limbaugh / Rosie O'Donnell Chris Christie / Camryn Manheim*
Oxypheric	*Winston Churchill / Orsen Welles Ella Fitzgerald / Gerry Spence*
Pargenic	*Burt Reynolds / Katey Segal Ron Perlman / Kirstey Alley*

<u>*Succinct Quote on Human Types*</u>

From Victor Rocine, who first described discrete body types around 1900.

"A type is an order of people that differentiates and distinguishes itself by a general and similar form, brain-formation, chemistry, structure, build, immunity, tendencies, predisposition, resemblance, skin-pigment, and type characteristics based on observation and analogy.

"Or, in other words, people of a given type are similar physically and like-minded as if they were brothers and sisters—that is what type means.

"Everything in nature is made according to plan. Man only discovers that plan and gives it a name. The zoologist has not made the animals—he has only described the plan adopted by the wonderful Creator, and named the classes, sub-classes, etc.

"How important type research will be to humanity, time alone will make known."

———

Prologue

The esteemed scientist J. J. Berzelius, discoverer of several chemical elements, inspired Victor Rocine to research body types and to investigate the correlation between types and their diseases. Around 1890-1910, Rocine privately published his original findings on the mineral basis of different body types, and this present book exists because of his brilliant insights.

For many years, I studied with Dr. Clifford Severn who had been a personal student of Victor Rocine on body types, naturopathy, herbology, iris analysis, diet, and nutritional healing methods. He had a successful career as a lecturer and healer, and was one of those rare athletes with complete muscle control over his body. I saw him under a spotlight at 85 years of age, contracting and rippling every individual muscle in his perfectly developed body. Field-Marshal Jan Smuts, the WWII South African Prime Minister, devoted a full chapter of his autobiography to how Severn's healing methods had saved his life. In the 1950's, *Life* magazine did a four-page spread on Severn and his family. Fame he had.

Another Rocine student I studied with, Dr. Bernard Jensen wrote of Rocine's body type research and nutritional methods in his privately published, *The Chemistry of Man*.

This book is deeply rooted in Rocine's original work, and with that of Herbert Shelton, M.D., Ph.D. (at Harvard University in the 1930's). I integrated their research with newer dietary and nervous system data along with celebrity examples of each type, hopefully, making this material easier to digest and more entertaining for the reader.

Gayelord Hauser, another Rocine student I knew, was a celebrated health book author. He wrote a popular book on Rocine's types in the 1940's, *Types and Temperaments;* reputedly, he also introduced yogurt to the western world.

This book exists because of Rocine's creative brilliance and original discoveries in natural healing.

▶ *Rocine: "The soul creates the body type."*

Rocine taught that the soul chooses a body type and brain to live in, thus presenting different experiences and life lessons to master. Why were *you* born the way you are?

That is something to think about, especially if it is true! What would your soul purpose be to live in a particular body type. I provide some thoughts on this issue in each type description and try to assess from my experience with your type the particular lessons of life presented therein.

Rocine was as brilliant in his way as an Abraham Lincoln, Michael Jordan, Michael Phelps, Tony Robbins, or a Daniel Day Lewis—all *calciferic* types—rare, leaders, innovative, brilliant, and highly intelligent in their different fields of endeavor.

Celebrity examples exist for most types, not a duplicate of you, but someone who has your essence in their body-mind individuality. Knowing your type allows you to become a better you!

The celebrity examples provide further help in identifying your body type.

▶ *Rocine's classic findings are the backbone of this book. Integrated with Sheldon's research and with other dietary and food issues including mental, emotional, and spiritual attributes,*

Many people take nutritional supplements and try different diets without a doctor's advice. If this is your choice, use common sense, listen to body responses, and discontinue any allergic reactions to foods or nutritional substances.

———

The Lipopheric
Body Type

"You may also have a physical or psychological feature not representative of your type such as height, weight, appearance, talent, weakness, strength, etc., due to biochemical errors, environmental influences, racial or cultural differences, and congenital or genetic issues. Nevertheless, the type identification of the average person is usually clear."

—Victor Rocine

Lipopheric Type Celebrity Examples

If you think this is your type, be sure to look at __on-line photographs__ of these examples. Look for general similarities to yourself. Note that sub-types cause the differences in appearance between members of the same type.

―――

POLITICS

Governor Chris Christie

RADIO/TV

Rush Limbaugh   Rosie O'Donnell
Ricki Lake

FILM/COMICS

Oliver Hardy
Sam Kinison   Jackie Gleason
Jack Black   Louie Anderson
Robbie Coltrane ("Harry Potter)
Camryn Manheim   Rebel Wilson

SPORTS

Jackie Gleason (in "The Hustler" he played another *lipopheric,* Minnesota Fats, the prior World pool champion)

ARTS

Fats Domino

HISTORY *(from Rocine)*

Henry VIII of England

[Note: I personally knew several members of this type, mostly men, which contributed to my understanding of them. Overall, they were intense, friendly, highly intelligent people.]

Read the type and if still confused, see *Appendix A,* for the personal type identification request from my website: *DrStenbeck.net*

———

Lipopheric Type Questionnaire

These questions describe the generic type, and not specifically you! If any question ever applied to you, then choose the True answer!

For Question 1 only:
A = True   *B = Maybe*   *C = Untrue*
15 points   *7 points*   *1 point*

1. Physically identify with celebrity example ____

Then...
A = True   *B = Maybe*   *C = Untrue*
5 points   *3 points*   *1 point*

---

2. Height is close to:
   Males: 5'8--6'4   Females: 5'0--5'9   ____
3. Usual weight is close to:
   Males: 180--400+ Females: 160--400+   ____
4. Body is fat or obese from an early age;
   weight very difficult to control   ____
5. Muscles large and strong   ____
6. Large body, small hands and feet   ____
7. Happy, jolly, optimistic   ____
8. Often vivacious, some plain-looking   ____
9. Large chest (medium hair growth in
   males); often a large bust   ____
10. Characteristic fat ball in cheeks   ____
11. Curved upper eyelids; thick lower lids   ____

12. Thick lower-half of the ears   _____
13. Wide lower-half of face; wide at the
    jaw angles   _____
14. High degree of intellectual courage   _____
15. Smaller top-head (heavy backhead)   _____
16. Dark or brown hair; back-head has a
    bald spot with aging (especially males)   _____
17. Lower eyelids thick with fat; "laughter
    lines" at outer corners of eyes   _____
18. Large lips: upper curves out; lower
    lip full in central part   _____
19. Chin broad; double or triple chins   _____
20. Gracious, courteous, pleasant;
    you attract people   _____
21. Skin white, creamy color; smooth,
    oily, velvet-like   _____
22. Communicate with emphatic head
    and hand gestures   _____
23. Very thick groin fat padding; thick
    and fat upper thighs   _____
24. Protruding fat abdomen in teens   _____
25. Arms often quite hairy; fatty wrists
    (with small bones)   _____
26. Weak joints, tendons, ligaments that
    are easily stressed   _____
27. Hands, feet are small; tapered fingers   _____
28. Are magnetic and inspirational   _____
29. Polite, gracious, courteous, able to
    speak truth without fear or regret; well-
    mannered,   _____
30. Are producers, communicators,
    collaborators, do-ers!   _____

31. Fun-loving, derisive sense of humor _____
32. Highly intelligent, many intellectuals _____
33. Loud voiced, provocative, have thought-out opinions _____
34. Are seeking or have found God _____
35. Are naturally aggressive _____
36. Show best side to strangers _____
37. Highly sentimental _____
38. Great love of nature _____
39. Love luxury, travel, "the good life" _____
40. Need to be around people _____
41. Very generous when have money _____
42. Scold and discipline others; able to speak truth without judgment _____
43. Have very high confidence _____
44. Inspire others with philosophy, knowledge, humor, friendliness, and intelligence _____
45. Limited degree of physical courage _____
46. Impress people at first meeting _____
47. Highly idealistic _____
48. Entrepreneurial ability, talent in sales and publicity _____
49. Have the courage to apologize for mistakes; limited physical courage _____
50. If crossed, may disown that person _____
51. Some have challenge with monogamy _____
52. Moderate will-power _____
53. Impatient and demanding _____
54. May sometimes rant and rave because of excessive passion and enthusiasm _____

55. Management, entrepreneur talents   _____
56. Excellent used car salesmen; easily
    stretch the truth   _____
57. Vigor, fervor, passions rule feelings   _____
58. Have little concentration for detail to
    be scientists; are found as lawyers
    and other professionals   _____
59. Are pleasant, happy, optimistic,
    humorous, and polite   _____
60. Desire to serve and help others   _____
61. Persuasive, pleasant, and magnetic   _____
62 Are assertive or aggressive   _____
63. Very strong ego; able to sell
    anything to anyone!   _____
64. Like to dominate and control others   _____
65. Impatient and demanding   _____
66. Great zest for life and communicate
    it to others   _____

Scoring

For question #1:
A response: give 15 points = _____
B response: give 7 points = _____
C response: give 1 points = _____

For questions #2—66:
A response: give 5 points = _____
B response: give 3 points = _____
C response: give 1 point = _____
Total of the above points = _____

Interpretation
153—295: PROBABLY Lipopheric Type

73—152: POSSIBLY Lipopheric type

<73: NOT Lipopheric type

The Lipopheric Type

Rocine: "Lipopheric means 'fat generating and holding.' You utilize more food <u>carbon, hydrogen and oxygen</u> than other types, these three elements making you a highly charismatic dynamo." You are highly intelligent,

---

The dormant and powerful energy within you usually manifests as action in your life. You serve others, while at the same time helping yourself! The legends around Henry VIII describe your type when out of control with most of the seven deadly sins! You are typically plump when young, and fat or obese as adults.

▶ *Rocine: "You are potentially the fattest of all types, absorbing and making fat from an early age because of insufficient oxygen in your tissues to convert hydrogen into water."*

Rush Limbaugh became a multi-millionaire by servicing a public need: if he did not believe what he was saying and doing his political fun and communication would never work. You inject self-belief into your work with great results.

▶ *Rush is such a perfect example of your appeal, power, brain, mind, and soul; whether one is conservative or not, call him genius or buffoon, his radio and public performances are a tour de force! And, he has taken command of his fat predisposition.*

Physical Similarity to Other Types

The *hydripheric* type (Rodney Dangerfield, Shelley Winters) is very commonly confused with the *lipopheric*; note the different head descriptions and the watery 'sloshy' fat of the *hydripheric* compared to your solid fat.

The fat *pallinomic* type (Ed McMann from "Star Search" and the prior "Tonight Show", and Attorney General Janet Reno) may be similar, but are fat muscle types.

The *oxypheric* type (Winston Churchill, Ella Fitzgerald) is more naturally expressive and out-going with a larger forehead and jaw.

The *barotic* type (Robin Williams, "Mrs. Doubtfire") is more rotund or obese, quiet, passive, and rare!

The *isogenic* type (Einstein, Ophrah Winfrey) is usually large and fleshy in females and older males, and is intellectual and philo-sophical.

––––––

Average Height and Weight

Males:	5'8--6'4	180--400+ pounds
Females:	5'0--5'9	160--400+ pounds

The fattest people in the world are of your type: some are 500 to 1000 pounds or more. You may maintain a moderately fleshy build into your late teens before gaining weight. Some of you are helped by having gastric by-pass surgery.

You already know something about this type from their public persona and appearance, whether from seeing them yourself or from the celebrity examples. Blend such insights with the type descriptions and the types of your family and friends to discern their presence in your midst!

––––––

Lipopheric Type Description

The type description represents how you appear in everyday society. You may have a sub-type that alters parts of this description.

Think of Governor Chris Christie, Rush Limbaugh, Jackie Gleason, Robert Morley, Ricki Lake, and Rosie O'Donnell as you read the descriptions. The central body is large, the hands and feet small. You are happy and jolly, attractive, vivacious or plain, but rarely shapely.

Head — The front of your top-head is prominent and may bulge. You have a relatively small head in comparison to body size; a few have a large head and are very tall. The back-head may be vertical.

▶ *Rocine: "Many of you have a small, upper back-head, and a heavy lower back-head. On profile, the distance from the top of the fore-head to the top of the back-head is often much less than in other fat types,"*

Hair — You have dark or brown hair with a bald spot starting at the back of your head.

Eyes — Your eyes are average-sized with blue, brown or hazel colors. Your upper eyelids are elevated and curved in the central area; the lower lid is thick with fat, and the eyebrows have a distinctive curve. "Laughter lines" appear around the outer corners of your sparkling and flirtatious eyes. You may show an intense whiteness to the eyes.

Ears — Your normal-sized ears have large lower ear lobes.

Nose — Your fleshy medium-sized nose has a thick nose-tip.

Face — A fleshy and broad chin has a deep dimple, with double or triple chins as you age. Your jaw-bones are not visible because of heavy fat deposition.

▶ *The lower half of your face is full, large and fatty at the angles of the jaw. A large fat-ball appears in the lower cheeks.*

The wide jaw angles, without fat pads, are also seen in the younger *desmogenic* type (Rocine: it denotes aggression, determination).

Mouth, Lips and Voice — The mouth is average, with shapely and even lips. The upper lip turns out at the inner edge while the lower lip is full in the central section and may curve outwards. The tongue is usually notably red.

Many females of this type have these lip characteristics.

▶ *You have a loud insistent, influential and outspoken voice (like the isogenic).*

A strident, loud, high-pitched, fervent voice with clear, confident, and positive enunciation typifies your verbal expression.

Teeth — You have white shapely teeth of normal size; decay problems develop as your health deteriorates.

Skin — Your smooth, oily, velvet-like textured skin usually has a white, light or creamy color.

Neck — A thick and fatty neck is typical.

Muscles — You have high strength and muscle building potential with many Olympic weightlifters being of your type. Your large body size precludes most sports other than American football, wrestling, and especially sumo at which you are world champions; but you are not as powerful as the *desmogenic* type.

▶ *A physician I knew weighed 250 pounds at age 20. A year later, after exercise and diet, he was rippling with muscles on a 180 pound body. Ten years later, he weighed 360 pounds. "I was just not up to the daily effort. The call of the food was too much," he said.*

Chest — Your chest is large and full with a pendulous bust. The lungs are usually very strong and healthy.

Back and Shoulders — Thick, strong, and plump back and shoulders are usual.

Hips and Abdomen — Have a fat and protruding abdomen by age 20.

▶ *Characteristically thick fat in the groin, inguinal areas and thighs.*

Arms and Legs — Your extremities are proportional to your height. Your arms tend to be quite hairy, but the bones of your wrist are small (like the *carboferic*) compared to your body size. Your hands and feet are usually small with tapered fingers.

▶ *Rocine: "Your hands are made for petting, not for striking hard blows."*

You have extremely thick, fat and strong thighs: you make great line-backers in football. If tall, your walk is heavy or light, and bouncy if shorter. An obese person with normal-sized thighs is often a fat *pallinomic* or an *isogenic* type.

Joints — Your joints, tendons, and ligaments are weak and vulnerable.

Weight — Your type is the heaviest of all types of people.

———

Lipopheric Personality Traits

If you are this type many, but not all, of the following characteristics are present—you may have overcome or moderated the negatives, but recognize that you once had several of them.

You may have any of the following traits:

- Confident, certain, desire to serve
- Have a mild and pleasant demeanor
- A limited degree of physical courage
- You actively seek a God relationship
- Love money, luxury, travel, the good life
- Use emphatic gestures in communicating
- Your feelings appear gushy, frantic, forceful
- Are producers, communicators, activists, do-ers
- Have a derisive sense of humor: many comedians
- Usually impress people at first sight and meeting

- Have enough courage to apologize for your errors
- A zim and zest for life that is easily communicated
- Changeable and moody: show best side to strangers
- Need and like people around all the time; are idealists
- Able to discipline others without anger: all is then forgiven
- Self-confidence is high, along with other self-positive feelings
- Vigor, fervor, and passion rule your feelings; when you want something you want it now
- Have gracious, courteous and pleasant manners: you attractive people, are exceedingly generous
- Are aggressive, dictatorial, festive, comedic, fun-loving, happy, optimistic, pleasant, magnetic, and polite
- Are highly intelligent, intellectual, sentimental, comfortable with yourself, and a great lover of nature
- You inspire and move others with your humor, philosophy, knowledge, friendliness and mental clarity

▶ *A lipopheric male, about 5'5" tall, in line at the bank spoke for us all. He yelled loudly, "Hey! Don't you have any service here? Everybody, let's move our accounts to another bank!" Needless to say service was immediately provided. The smile on his face reflected his enjoyment at the attention to his personal power!*

―――

Potential Challenges

You may have evolved from or not experienced these general challenges, so don't dwell on them.

- May rant and rave sometimes
- Haughty, impatient, demanding, ego-centric
- Excellent salesperson: able to stretch the truth
- Excellent actors: may use this talent to influence others
- May have difficulty with monogamy (unless spiritually evolved)
- Will-power and concentration weak: long term projects tire you
- Need to influence and dominate people: if you cannot, that person may be discarded

―――

Lipopheric Stress Management

You have strong mental and emotional stress prevention providing a good ability not to internalize stress into your body. (If needing help managing these stresses, see my prior books.)

———

Love

You are romantic, expressive, playful, and kind. The *atrophic, calciferic, exesthesic or neurogenic* types attract you—your physical opposites. You make excellent mates. Your intellect is so strong that you are able to think through and resolve any relationship problem.

———

Talents and Vocations

Abilities — *Management, entrepreneur, public speaking, public service professions, publicity, religion, transport, sales*

You are happiest when using your voice in radio, TV, sales, lecturing, influencing others, etc.; are born to sales. You have management abilities, but not in the same class as the *myogenic, desmogenic, nitropheric, and calciferic* types. Some of you may become intuitives, psychics, and healers (especially females).

▶ *I have known, or observed you as physicians, cooks, lawyers, waiters, comics, psychics, restaurant managers, super-salesmen, rock singers, and in successful businesses.*

The type information cannot predict what or who you will become, but you are capable of bringing a creative excellence or brilliance to whatever you do in life.

Inabilities — *Scientific, physical labor*

You rarely have the concentration and patience for detail to be scientists, although because of your high intelligence you are found as physicians, lawyers, and other professionals.

———

Acid/Alkaline Factor

For your health and healing, your nervous system genetics require a specific ratio of acid to alkaline foods. You are born with **intermediate** dominance (between *parasympathetic* and *sympathetic*), and need *balanced* acid and alkaline-ash food intake. (Ash refers to the minerals left in your body after metabolizing foods.) You may indulge in both food classes. Construct this approximate ratio of food selections:

> *50% Fruits, salads, vegetables*
> *50% Proteins, carbohydrates*

▶ *Approximate your food ratios. On any particular day, it does not matter if one meal is mostly alkaline and another mostly acid—just try to balance it out for the day! If you make a mistake, try again tomorrow. It is a subjective call that you make, as what you do over weeks and months makes the difference to your health.*

Lipopheric Spiritual Factor

Skip this paragraph if uninterested in a philosophical perspective on your type!

▶ *Rocine: "The soul chooses the body type."*

If as souls, we choose the brain and body type to spend a lifetime in, it could be to learn certain spiritual lessons related to perfecting ourselves, and our humanity, in God's eyes. What lessons does the type bring you? Only you can really decide what those lessons are. You know your weaknesses, faults, and behaviors towards others. You know things about yourself that Victor Rocine could never get from his research subjects when he first wrote about types. So search your mind for the answers.

Each discrete type has challenges of life lessons, spiritual goals, etc., and some of yours may be:

Faith — Your faith is dependent on what your huge rational brain can make of God and religion. God is a very hard sell for you.

Temper — You have a short fuse: work on becoming more patient.

Arrogance — You are superior to many people, but not in God's eyes: moderate your huge ego!

Low Will-power — This problem may interfere with your success: seek out mind-control, hypnosis, etc.

Ego-Centric — Because of your strong ego you need to command and dominate others: forgive our lesser brains and work on your humility!

———

Health Problems

When sick, you commonly experience health problems or diseases in any of the following organs and tissues:

Liver — The liver readily becomes toxic.

Intestines — The intestines are vulnerable to disease.

Circulatory System — This system is vulnerable to disease.

Fatty Infiltrations — Disease comes from fatty infiltration and nerve obstruction in the heart, liver, spleen, and brain, etc.

———

A Lipopheric Story...

Pat, 280 pounds, had been fat since early childhood and was not really expecting any help with that problem. His complaints were around an enlarged heart, high blood pressure, kidney, and other problems—actually a "global" body problem due to fat. He hated exercise and did not attempt it.

Dietary evaluation showed he was eating sensibly, but he was eating excessive hydrogen foods: alcohol, almonds, avocado, breads, celery, cereals, cocoa, cheese, corn, eggs, head lettuce, meats, poultry, and watermelon. He was also deficient in potassium and calcium foods needed for his type: kelp, brewers yeast, turnip greens, sunflower seeds, parsley, corn tortillas, dandelion greens, raisins, and Brazil nuts.

Pat made these dietary changes, took the herbs indicated for his type, and his weight and organ health steadily improved. He achieved 180 pounds and was motivated to begin exercising!

———

Lipopheric Type Mineral Needs

Apply this mineral data to the diet following the Fat type descriptions.

Excessive Foods:
- *Carbon (simple carbohydrates)*
- *Hydrogen*
- *Oxygen*
- *Sodium (salted, junk)*

Deficient Foods:
- *Trace Minerals*
- *Potassium*
- *Sodium (unsalted, non-junk)*
- *Hot Citrus Drinks, Shellfish Broths*

These deficient minerals are common deficiencies in your type, and predispose you to ill-health.
If ill, be sure to use these lists with your daily food intake. If not ill, eat from the food lists 3-4 days weekly for health maintenance.
All food lists are in descending order of concentration and value to you; choose servings of foods in the upper half of each list first! One serving is ½ cup.

Note - The above recommendations are for the generic type. Additionally, you may need from a holistic healer or nutritionist, something more specific for your individuality.

Lipopheric Excessive Foods –

Carbon is the basis of all life, and is excessive in all people who become fat. It is excessive in your type, so minimize your intake of simple carbohydrates: white and brown sugars, high fructose corn syrup, honey, maple syrup, molasses, jellies, candy, ice cream, soda drinks.

Instead, eat complex carbohydrates: yams, potatoes, squash, pumpkin, corn, lentils, peas, beans, green vegetables, grains (and foods made from them).

Hydrogen is excessive in your type, contributing to obesity and water-logging of your tissues.

Oxygen is excessive (along with iron and potassium), and is important in the metabolism of muscles, red blood cells, and all cells. In excess it promotes unrealistic enthusiasm in this type.

Sodium from salted junk foods is excessive in your tissues. To preserve your health and weight control you should avoid junk foods, and fulfill your sodium needs from the food list without using the salt shaker (but potassium salt is appropriate.) Along with potassium, food sodium is vital for normalizing your calcium metabolism and for preventing calcium deposits in your tissues and joints.

————

Deficient Foods –

In illness or disease, it is important to correct these deficiencies.

Trace minerals easily become deficient in your type due to emotional stress or poor digestion and absorption.

Potassium is often deficient in your type. It is a dominant element in your tissues and is concentrated in and vital to the health of your muscles, heart, brain, and all cells. If ill or diseased, potassium foods and supplements are probably a significant healing factor.

Sodium as unsalted non-junk foods is deficient in your tissues.

Hot citrus drinks and shellfish broths are helpful to your health, healing, and weight loss.

————

<u>*Minimize*</u>

Excessive Foods

Carbon, Hydrogen, Oxygen:
0-1 servings/week

All fats and fatty foods, carbohydrates, starches, grains, breads, sweet fruits, oils, blackberries, meats, liver, head lettuce, asparagus, whole grain cereals and breads, dried fruits, prunes, legumes, pumpkin, watermelon, celery, alcohol, almonds, avocado, butter, cereals, chocolate, cookies, pies, etc., all white sugar foods, cocoa, coconuts, cheeses, corn, cream.

Sodium (salted, junk): *0-1 servings/week*

Salt, all fast foods, packaged foods, canned and frozen foods, soy sauce, all preserved meats (cured, smoked, canned and luncheon meats), sauces (barbecue, catsup, etc.), dill pickles, sauerkraut, bouillon cubes, peanut butter, potato chips, etc., salted nuts, crackers, packaged soups, processed cheeses, commercial salad dressings, meat tenderizers.

Note: If you must eat anything on the above lists, keep it down to ½ cup, 0-1 times weekly!

Eat

Deficient Foods

Trace Minerals: *1-2 servings/day*
*Swiss and goat cheese, raw cabbage,
cartilaginous broth, Irish moss, clams
and shellfish broths, lean meats, dark green
leafy vegetables, garlic, mushrooms, spinach.*

Potassium: *1-2 servings/day*

*Dulse, kelp, brewer's yeast, rice bran, sunflower
seeds, parsley, corn tortillas, dandelion greens,
raisins, sesame seeds, rice polish, brazil nuts.*

Sodium (unsalted, non-junk):
1-2 servings/day

*Kelp, cheese, gizzard, buttermilk, lentils, Swiss
chard, beets and greens, eggs, cod, coconut, salt
water fish, spinach, lamb, turkey, pistachio and
sesame (unsalted), okra, watercress, milk.*

Hot Citrus Drinks:

*Rocine recommended you drink liberally of hot
citrus drinks for your healing and weight loss.
Note: Eat any other healthy foods you desire,
but be sure to include the type food suggestions in
your daily choices.*

Lipopheric Nutritional Supplements

- **Multi-Vitamins-Minerals**
  [Take all supplements with food]
  — 2 capsules/day
- **Potassium** *— 99 mg/day with food*

- **Kelp** *— 4 tablets/ twice daily*
- **Manganese** *— 50 mg/day with food*

- **Herbs** *—*
  Brain detox – Gingko or Dong Quai
  Organ detox – Saw Palmetto or Milk
  Thistle
  (Take one capsule, twice daily for one
  month; then one, three times weekly.)

- **Evening Primrose or Flaxseed**
  Oil *— 1 soft-gel/day with food*

- **Other** *— Chlorophyll, blue-green algae,*
  green magma, spirulina, alfalfa, or other
  source. (Take as directed: three times/week)
  Note: Be sure to take these supplements if
  you have ill-health. If you are in good
  health, take them at least 3-4times/week.

Important Lipopheric Health Concerns

Your nervous system genetics require the *Fat* type Food Guide for health, and any carnivorous cravings are normal and healthy for you. After about age 40, have three flesh days weekly, and vegetarian the other days. Minimize red meats.

▶ *Rocine: "Your diseases are caused by tissue fat-building, uncontrolled appetite and fat generation, from which dangerous diseases may quickly follow. You should avoid cold drinks, and drink hot citrus drinks and shellfish broths instead."*

LIPOPHERIC FOOD GUIDE

Aim for -

50% Proteins, carbohydrates
50% Fruits, salads, vegetables
and
50% Raw food diet
50% Cooked foods

Take the recommended supplements.
Follow Rocine's advice.

Lipopheric Weight Loss

Your body absorbs excessive fat from an early age, and you have great difficulty in losing it. Follow the diet and you will make good progress. Give yourself permission to exercise! It is essential for your fat burning.

- *Drink,* mostly, warm or hot citrus juices and clam or shellfish broths over choosing water!
- *Avoid* all the excessive foods (see list)
- *Protein* drink in citrus juice daily, about 25-30 grams
- *Eat* your body type deficient mineral foods daily
- *Follow* your *Lipopheric Guide (as above)*
- *Exercise*: your body type requires only moderate daily exercise (like walking or swimming)
- *Simple sugars*: stop all white table sugar and high-fructose corn syrup and drinks containing these sugars
- *Instead of diet pills,* you need glucomanin supplements that swell and take up space in the stomach thus preventing over-eating
- *If hypoglycemic* (low blood sugar, fatigue, depression, etc.), which stops fat loss and usually initiates more fat production, it is vital to deal with this problem: take

pantothenic acid, 500 mg/twice daily with food (see my earlier books to resolve this problem)

- *Calories:* As with any dietary approach, calories in must be *less than* calories out! Most markets sell a calorie booklet; make notes of your daily intake, and in most instances keep it under about 1500-1800 calories/day

-----

Fat Types
General Food Guide

---

*(An Intermediate Guide between
Carnivores and Vegetarians)*

Important Note

———

The Food Guide addresses the <u>Acid-Alkaline</u> aspect of your food intake, along with the <u>Type Mineral</u> factor presented throughout this book. It does <u>not</u> necessarily address calories or other dietary factors that may be pertinent to your personal health needs whether medical or appropriate for some other dietary need. So use your common sense and just include the factors described here with whatever healthy dietary choices you usually make.

For other nutrient information, consult with nutritional books or with holistic nutritional doctors. In this regard, I particularly recommend the advice of Andrew Weil, M.D.

———

Fat Types
General Food Guide

This chapter presents an <u>Intermediate</u> Food Guide, balanced between the Muscle types (carnivores) and the Thin types (vegetarians). Superimpose the individual type mineral and other information from your type chapter into this Food Guide (which is not for the pargenic type.)

———

Meat/Flesh Intake

Generally, animal protein is acceptable and needed in your diet: red meat should be limited to once weekly or less, while lamb and fish or poultry are excellent in moderation. If this diet is similar to what you are already eating, but you have health problems because of a history of excess acid-ash food intake being so common, then:

- Decrease your carbohydrate and protein intake by about one-third
- Increase your fruit, salad and vegetable intake by about one-third
- Consult with a holistic doctor, preferably one versed in nutritional and emotional evaluation

———

Over-Acid or Over-Alkaline?

Just as a log of wood burned in your fireplace leaves a mineral-ash, food ash refers to the minerals remaining after metabolizing foods in your tissues:

- Fruits and vegetables **alkalinize** tissues
- Proteins and carbohydrates **acidify** tissues

You are usually over-acid due to:

- Accumulated metabolic waste-acids
- Deficient fruit, salad and vegetable intake
- Excessive protein and carbohydrate intake

You need to estimate the ratio of foods you are eating: generally, eat the following *approximate* ratio of foods for your health:

50% *Alkaline-ash* foods (fruits, salads, vegetables)
50% *Acid-ash* foods (complex carbohydrates like starches, grains, cereals, breads, flour products; and proteins)

Approximate your food ratios. On any particular day it does not matter if one meal is mostly alkaline, and another is acid—just try to balance it out for the day! If you make a mistake, forget it and try again tomorrow. It is a subjective call that you make. It is what you do over weeks and months that makes the difference to your health—not on any few days.

The net result is that the Fat types require the plan presented in this chapter for health restoration.

[The following chart shows the fat types, their acid-alkaline reactions, and the percentage of raw foods needed for their healing.]

Fat Types

Acid/Alkaline Genetics   Dietary-Ash and Raw Food Needs

———

This chart shows the Rocine types, their acid or alkaline food needs, and the percentage of raw foods needed for your health and healing.

BODY TYPE	ACID/ALKALINE GENETICS	% DIET ASH	% RAW FOODS
Barotic	*Intermediate*	*50:50*	*50*
Carboferic	*Intermediate*	*50:50*	*50*
Hydripheric	*Intermediate*	*50:50*	*30*
Isogenic	*Intermediate*	*50:50*	*30*
Lipopheric	*Intermediate*	*50:50*	*50*
Oxypheric	*Intermediate*	*50:50*	*50*
Pargenic	*Acid*	*70% alkaline*	*30*

Note that the above percentages will vary depending on aging and the health of individual types.

Notes

- Never eat foods you are allergic to, no matter what I recommend here; if you suspect allergy to a suggested food, eliminate it.

- Minimize your white sugar and alcohol intake.

- Eat the right foods most of the time and the diet will help you; you do not have to live out of a health food store (although such foods are healthier).

- All food lists are in descending order of concentration and value to you as a mineral source; whenever possible, choose foods in the upper half of each list first! One serving is ½ cup.

- If desired, you may interchange lunches for dinners.

- Avoid all junk foods, white sugar, foods with added sugar, and high fructose corn syrup

———

General Food Guide

Breakfasts

[Superimpose the nutritional information from your

EGGS (1-2) with lettuce, tomato, whole grain toast — 1-3 times/week; or

FRUIT SALAD, fresh with citrus fruit and a protein source (low-sugar yogurt, kefir, milk, cottage cheese, cheese, seeds or nuts) — 2-4 times/week; or

COOKED CEREALS, fruit, seeds, whole grain, and nuts — 2-5 times/week; or

OTHER — 0-1 times/week

Eat unlimited fruit, salads, vegetables, with seeds/nuts for snacks. Wheat is a common allergy: avoid white and wheat breads; eat rye, sour dough, or oat breads instead

* * *

DAILY LIQUIDS

Pure water — as desired (except Hydripheric type)
Fruit and vegetable juices — 0-2 cups
Coffee, caffeine teas — 0-2 cups

[Include selections from your type mineral needs with each meal.]

Lunches

SALADS, mixed green, and 2-4 oz., of protein (fish, poultry, egg, cheese, tofu, seeds or nuts, etc.) [Dressings: use canola or olive oil* and vinegar; or low-fat/calorie dressing] — 2-4 times/week; or

VEGETABLES (steamed) with salad, and yogurt, or cottage cheese (or other breakfast proteins) — 1-2 times/week; or

FRUIT SALAD (see breakfast) — 0-1 times/week

SANDWICH, whole grains with a non-flesh protein (egg, tofu, cheese, etc.) — 1-3 times/week; or

POULTRY, FISH, 3-4 oz., with a mixed green salad and/or steamed vegetables (or as a sandwich) — 1-2 times/week; or

OTHER — 0-1 times/week

* Other oils less ideal; soybean is common allergen; minimize commercial dressings

[Include selections from your type mineral needs with each meal.]

Dinners

LEAN POULTRY OR FISH (4-6 oz.)
— 2-4 times/week

PASTA, PROTEIN (as above)
—1-3 times/week

VEGETARIAN MEAL, including legumes, tofu,
cheese, cottage cheese, seeds or nuts, egg, etc.
—2-4 times/week

LEAN BEEF (4-6 oz.) — 0-2 times/month

OTHER — 0-2 times/week

Take all of the above with: mixed green salad,
dressing (as before), and/or vegetables (steamed are
best).

DESSERTS

Fruits, fresh — as desired
Low-sugar, healthy desserts —0-3 times/week

If you have blood fat problems, cholesterol or
triglycerides, eliminate all beef from your diet, and
see my earlier books.

Eat fruit, unlimited salads and vegetables with
seeds/nuts, low-sugar yogurt for snacks.

[Include selections from your type mineral
needs with each meal.]

Fat Types Notes

Do not eat flesh everyday: have it on alternate days only. For munchies, have low calorie items like celery and other vegetables, along with yogurt and cottage cheese, etc. Some of you abuse your beef and red meat intake, perhaps several times weekly—this is a false craving; use your will to combat it if you want to be healthier!

Steamed Vegetables —Minerals are lost in the boiling of vegetables; best is steaming or wok cooking.

Minimize Foods — Only eat them 0-1 times/week! Be sure to eat the recommended foods to help your healing;

Food Combinations —Eating proteins at the same meal with starches often results in indigestion, gas or constipation (along with low blood sugar and making fat). Watch how this inharmonious food combination may be affecting you.

Minimize —

- All fatty foods
- Milk and dairy foods (unless otherwise noted)
- Commercial, sugared, and fatty salad dressings

- Beef, sugar, wines, alcohol, coffee, white sugar, red meats, and processed meats

Vegetarian Proteins — If you choose to be vegetarian, it will help your health after middle-age; because you have semi-carnivorous genes be sure to take a protein supplement of 20-30 grams/day (e.g., soy or egg-white powder in juice).

Healthy Weight — Invariably you hold excessive weight, and in addition to body type factors there may be a medical problem behind your fat storage. By eating according to your body type, you slowly and naturally lose excess weight! Accumulating evidence indicts high-fructose corn syrup as a major cause of increased weight and obesity. Avoid it!

You have a sluggish fat-burning metabolism, and may have an under-active adrenal, thyroid, or pituitary gland resulting in hypoglycemia, and in this instance may need the services of a holistic doctor *(see Appendix* and my earlier books).

In Conclusion

I hope you have enjoyed reading this book. You should now know your body type and have learned some valuable information about how to be a healthier you! Do not forget my previous books on healing yourself.

If you desire further help or information with your body type or health from a holistic viewpoint, email me from page one of my web page:
Dr.Stenbeck.net

Good health and good luck!

———

Appendix

Brief Extracts from
<u>The 22 Unique Body Types</u>

Appendix A

Types
(Brief extract)

Type comes from 'typus' meaning an image or impression, the study of types being called typology.

▶ *Rocine: "A combination of mental and structural features is consistently found in people of the same type."*

Rocine wrote that all types are a mixture of positive and negative qualities. He based his work on the biochemical individuality of our *mineral* absorption and utilization. Of course, all minerals are absorbed, but he postulated that different types of people *selectively* absorb certain minerals, to a greater or lesser extent, requiring specific mineral foods for their enhanced health and healing.

▶ *The type information cannot predict what or who you will become, or how successful or not, but your type is capable of bringing a creative excellence to whatever you do in life. If your type has negative qualities that you disagree with, remember that they are only tendencies and may or may not manifest in you.*

This book enlarges on Rocine's premise (early 1900's), integrated with the later research of Herbert Sheldon, M.D., Ph.D., at Harvard University (1930's), along with my fifty years of observations and experience with this subject.

Comparing your shared physical (and sometimes psychological) descriptions with the Celebrity Lists further assists the identification of your type. It is not that you will look exactly like, or be a twin to, any particular celebrity. Look closely at a celebrity's features: face, profile, height, weight, head, etc. If you know something about their talents, beliefs, success and failure spheres, health and weight challenges, attitudes and behaviors, etc., then you get clues as to what your type may be.

————

Understanding Types and Sub-Types

Each of us has a clearly discernible dominant type. Visualize the celebrity examples from movies, politics, sports, the arts and public life, and try to identify with their physical features. Look for similar features, remembering that you will not recognize all attributes in yourself. You are not looking for your twin!

The sub-type issue is the main reason people of the same major type can look so different. Remember that a type description does not characterize you exactly, but depicts your individual variant of a type.

▶ *The type questionnaire pinpoints the major features of that type: if the celebrity examples are unhelpful, you may be an unusual variant (in which case ignore the celebrity issue and give yourself 7 points on Question 1).*

———

Minerals

Minerals are essential life nutrients that accelerate enzyme and chemical reactions and provide a basis for your body typing. Although found in all tissues, different minerals tend to be concentrated in certain organs, their presence or absence contributing to the healing of such tissues; e.g., zinc accelerates prostate healing; calcium and manganese promote bone, joint and connective tissue healing.

Specific foods nurture each type, some people needing meats for their health others needing a vegetarian diet. A high potassium diet nurtures one person, while another needs high sulfur, calcium, zinc, or another mineral.

Mineral Digestion and Absorption

Compared to vitamins, minerals are *difficult* to digest, absorb, and utilize. In people with strong digestive systems, this aspect may not be important. The following factors should be in place for optimal mineral metabolism:

1. Stomach Hydrochloric Acid Production
2. Parathyroid Hormone Balance
3. Organ Toxic Metal and Chemical Removal
   [See details in The 22 Unique Body Types.*]*

Total Body Healing

Note that from a holistic healing perspective, in addition to minerals and type information, the following healing factors are necessary:

> *Nutrient Balance*
> *Mental Balance*
> *Emotional Balance*
> *Spiritual Balance*
> *Detoxifying Integrity*

The above factors are all important to your total healing especially if you are interested in self-healing (see my earlier books).

Appendix B

Researchers
(Brief extract)

The predominant workers in this area of human individuality from around 1880's to the 1960's are Herbert Sheldon, M.D., Ph.D., Roger Williams, Ph.D., and Victor Rocine, D.Sc.

Much information on Sheldon's research exists on-line and in medical psychology libraries; for interested readers there are other lines of research published in the last century. This present book is primarily about Rocine's body types.

Herbert Sheldon M.D., Ph.D.

In contrast to Rocine, Sheldon at Harvard University in the 1930's was trained in the scientific method and did painstaking research and publishing on human individuality. In comparing his findings with Rocine's work, a direct putative correlation is visible.

Roger J. Williams, Ph.D.

Another significant researcher in human individuality is the renowned scientist and biochemist, Roger J. Williams. He demonstrated that different people have varying levels of nutrients, enzymes, and other metabolic chemicals in their bloodstreams.

▶ *Williams's research firmly expands on the premise of individual nutritional needs in human beings. If interested in his research, I highly recommend his book <u>Biochemial Individuality</u>.*

Victor Rocine, D.Sc.

Note that when a negative feature is indicated, say neurotic tendencies, all members of the type are <u>not</u> that way; it is a type tendency reported by Rocine.

Rocine studied type-related diseases finding links between mineral and dietary factors with individual types and their diseases. In each body type, one or more dominant minerals are preferentially absorbed and utilized over other minerals.

He recognized discrete body types from their physical appearance finding genetically based mineral dominance to be the determining feature. He also correlated their physical features with psychological characteristics.

———

Genetics, Types, and Diet
(Brief extract)

This section deals with how nervous system genetics helps determine your eating choices for health: you are either born to be a predominant meat eater, a partial or complete vegetarian, or something between the two. The genetic factor determining this dietary aspect is the *sympathetic and parasympathetic* components of your central nervous system. This represents a basic factor in eating for health.

This chapter helps you understand your dietary inheritance, although instinctively, you may already have arrived there!

- If born **sympathetic** dominant you are *genetically acid*, desiring a predominantly *vegetarian* diet for your health (about 70% fruit, salad, vegetables to 30% proteins and carbohydrates).

- If born **parasympathetic** dominant you are *genetically alkaline*, desiring a predominantly *carnivorous* diet for your health (about 70% proteins, carbohydrates to 30% fruits, salads, vegetables). Few of you ever choose to become vegetarian because of the difficulty in satisfying your protein needs without meats.

- If born ***intermediate*** dominant you may eat food groups with little concern for the acid/alkaline factor. However, after age 40, you need a semi-vegetarian diet for healthy eating.

———

Chart of Relative Nervous System Dominance

In the following Chart, if you relate to many of the symptoms on one side you probably have that nervous system dominance; relating to both sides indicates *Intermediate* dominance.

If Vegetarian (Over-acid) --
> *Eat 70% fruits, salads, vegetables*
> *And 30% proteins, carbohydrates*

If Carnivore (Over-alkaline) --
> *Eat 70% proteins, carbohydrates*
> *And 30% fruits, salads, vegetables*

If Intermediate --
> *Eat 50:50 of acid and alkaline-ash foods*

Make an *approximate* estimate of your daily acid and alkaline food intake (such ratios varying from type to type).

———

Symptoms of Relative Genetic Dominance

Vegetarians (Over-acid)	*Carnivores* (Over-alkaline)
Sympathetic Dominance	*Parasympathetic Dominance*
little or no flesh desire	desire flesh
easily constipated	rarely constipated
slow digestion	fast digestion
easily dehydrated	not dehydrated
strong thirst	low thirst
pale face	flushed face
high pulse after food	slow pulse after food
easy gag reflex	slow gag reflex
cool dry skin	moist warm skin
nervous stomach	calm stomach
little eyelid blinking	much blinking
nervous tendency	mostly calm
slower healing	faster healing
low oxygen-uptake	good oxygen-uptake
easily breathless	seldom breathless
insomnia common	sleep easier
few muscle cramps	some night cramps
calcium deposits rare	get calcium deposits

Appendix D

*Help Identifying your Body Type with **Dr. Stenbeck***

If you desire help in identifying your body type, follow these instructions, and answer the questionnaire. For further information and fees, send me an email from page one of the website:

DrStenbeck.net

First name: _____

Country of birth: _____

Upload photos and send to the above website:

■ Head and shoulders: front and side views

■ Full body: front and side views

■ Also 1-2 teenage views

■ If possible, casual photos of mother, father, siblings

MY TYPE CLASS MAY BE: _____

   (Thin, Muscle, or Fat)

AGE - _____

HEIGHT - _____ feet/inches

MY WEIGHT - _____ pounds

   Heaviest at age: _____

- Lightest as adult: _____

- Estimate age 15: _____

VISION - Excellent Average   Poor:

HAIR -   Natural color: _____

     - Thin/thick?   _____

     - balding?   _____

SKIN - Quality: _____

     - History of acne, boils, other:

_____

_____

TEETH   - Strong   Weak   Dentures

       - Cavity history: Many   Moderate   Few

MUSCLES - Strong   Average   Weak

     Sports played _____

JOINTS   - Strong   Average   Weak

HEALTH - Childhood diseases?

_____

_____

- Adult diseases?

_____

AVERAGE DIET

- Beef _____ (times/week)

- Poultry _____ (times/week)

- Fish _____ (times/week)

- Eggs _____ (times/week)

- Water _____ (glasses/day):

- Vegetarian? Vegan? _____

- Other? _____

- Did your childhood diet differ? _____

The above will help me know who you are! I will send you a follow-up questionnaire for further help in identifying your body type.

Appendix E

On-line Health Consultation with Dr. Stenbeck

For further information, or to comment on this book, or to receive a response on any health issue from a holistic viewpoint, send an email inquiry from page one of my website:

DrStenbeck.net

Following that, I will suggest further healing needs, which we may pursue with an on-line consult.

———

Appendix F

Notes

See my book *The 22 Unique Body Types,* available at the usual online source, for further information and details on all of the 22 Types. The Appendix in that book has further information about:

Mineral Functions and Food Sources

Further Reading

―――――